T0128691

I DO IT THE S.A.F.E. WAY

How I Stay Ahead of Parkinson's Disease,
Revised Edition

TOM S. GATSES

iUniverse, Inc.
Bloomington

I Do It the S.A.F.E. Way
How I Stay Ahead of Parkinson's Disease, Revised Edition

iUniverse books may be ordered through booksellers or by contacting:

iUniverse
1663 Liberty Drive
Bloomington, IN 47403
www.iuniverse.com
1-800-Authors (1-800-288-4677)

ISBN: 978-1-4697-7373-5 (sc)
ISBN: 978-1-4697-7374-2 (ebk)

Printed in the United States of America

iUniverse rev. date: 02/01/2012

I dedicate this book to all caretakers around the world. Whatever illness you may have—Parkinson's, cancer, MS, etc.—you might rely on caretakers who take the time away from their daily living to take care of people with severe disabilities. These caretakers should be recognized and praised for sacrificing themselves to make life easier for people with all types of debilitating diseases. God bless each and every one of you.

Contents

The Meaning of S.A.F.E.

S. Support—A strong system of support from family, friends, and doctors is essential. When you have support, you tend to try harder and feel better about yourself.

A. Attitude—You must have a strong and positive attitude. Never feel like you will not get better; feel positive, and remember, a good attitude is half the battle.

F. Faith—You must believe in yourself and in God. A strong faith can overcome anything.

E. Exercise—It is mandatory in your everyday living. It is very important to exercise a minimum of one hour per day. The benefits you will achieve from exercising will have a tremendous impact on your life.

You have the power and knowledge to add this simple concept, S.A.F.E., to your everyday life. You will feel healthier, look better, and possibly live longer. I wrote this book with the hope of inspiring and motivating people of all ages who have Parkinson's or any other debilitating disease. There are many books on Parkinson's disease, but I have made this book very easy to read and understand. If you are among the many who are currently struggling with this illness, I hope that, after you read this book, your quality of life will improve dramatically.

Preface

In this short but powerful book, I will show you how to accomplish all that you thought you could never do. I will explain Parkinson's and help you understand how to live with and stay ahead of Parkinson's disease—or any other ailments you may have.

I am on my thirteenth year of living with Parkinson's. I have learned to accept and live with it. I believe that the way I cope with my disease, using my S.A.F.E. method, I can beat Parkinson's or stay way ahead of it.

You will not find a better book on having a positive attitude. It is so easy to read and easy to understand. This book is enjoyable, interesting, educational, at times emotional, and definitely inspiring. After reading my book, I'm sure that you will discover that it has had an impact on your life. It will even be a useful tool for people with other debilitating diseases.

My book explains how I fight Parkinson's through support, attitude, faith, and exercise. Most of all, you will see how I treat Parkinson's through combat. I think I have the best attitude possible. This is how I feel. Some people may not agree with the way I fight this disease; that's fine! You deal with it your way, and I'll deal with it my way. At least I know that my way is working for me.

Acknowledgments

My wife, Jennie, is my backbone. Without her strength and support, I would probably be in a wheelchair by now. Jennie spent days trying to find the best neurologist for me. During our visits, she would always have paper and pencil handy because she had many questions that she had to have answered and explained. My wife is a strong person; she not only stands behind me, she pushes me to do whatever it takes to fight this dreaded disease.

My children have always had the greatest respect for me. When they learned of this diagnosis, they felt helpless. They tried to console and encourage me. We are a very close and emotional family, and my children know how much I have always liked to exercise and keep active. When we are all together to discuss my disease, they remind me to never stop doing what I love and enjoy most in life—exercising.

I have a great rapport with my daughter and sons. We joke, laugh, play, and even cry together. We are always there for one another, no matter what. I thank my family for all that they have given me so far.

Support

A person with an illness needs support, especially from his family.

Support gives you a feeling that you're wanted, and it builds your confidence and self-esteem. When you have no support, you tend to give up on yourself, and you begin to deteriorate. That's because you think no one cares about you.

We all must make it our priority to give support to those in need.

Attitude

Attitude plays a major role in acceptance of your disease.

How you treat your disease is very important. Do you accept what you have? Or are you in denial, letting yourself wither away and die? Don't feel sorry for yourself; think positive. When you worry about your disease, your condition may progress to a more serious level. You cannot change what has happened to you, but you can keep it from progressing.

I myself have a strong positive attitude toward my illness. I accept what I have and deal with it to the best of my abilities.

Faith

It has been said that faith can move mountains.

If you are a believer, faith can do that and much more. You must have faith in yourself and in God. Believe that someday soon a cure will be found for your illness. This belief will strengthen you by meeting your spiritual needs—and it might keep you from progressing to another stage. Praying helps especially when you feel like you want to talk to God. Be an optimist and think positive. You will be at peace with yourself and with everyone else.

Father Chris Kerhulas of Saint Basil's Greek Orthodox Church and the Very Reverend Father Timothy G. Bakakos Archimandrite of Assumption Greek Orthodox Church, both in Chicago, have helped me to believe in God and keep my faith. Without their support and confidence in me, I would have had a much harder time living with my Parkinson's disease. Their prayers for me to cope with my illness have been answered; I am doing exceptionally well. When I am down, all I have to do is call on either of them, and they will be there for me. They will always be with me, wherever I go and in my prayers. I am deeply grateful to them both for their wisdom and spiritual strength.

Exercise

Exercising is imperative in all stages of life.

Regardless of what illness you have, there are many exercises that you can do. Exercise will definitely make you feel better, and it might stop your illness from progressing. The stronger you are, the better chance you have of combating your sickness. Exercise strengthens muscles and makes your bones stronger. It will give you a sense of security and confidence as you fight your disease. The weak perish while the strong survive.

. When you fight, you try to win. When you don't fight, you are giving in to your illness, and the consequences may be fatal. No one can force you to exercise, but forcing yourself may keep you alive long enough that a cure can be found. Don't exercise to impress others; exercise for your life. It's your body.

What Is Parkinson's Disease?

I have read many definitions of Parkinson's disease. The best and easiest to understand defines it as a medical condition characterized by tremors, muscular stiffness, and slow movement caused by a brain disease of unknown origin. Dopamine, a chemical that is found in your brain, allows smooth, coordinated function of the body's muscles and movement. When approximately 80 percent of the dopamine-producing cells are damaged, the symptoms of Parkinsonism—a group of movement disorders with similar characteristics—appear.

Who Can Get Parkinson's Disease?

Anyone can get this debilitating disease. One person out of every thousand will eventually get Parkinson's disease. Usually, the signs of Parkinson's appear after the age of fifty, but many people are diagnosed at an earlier age. As you get older, your chances of getting this disease increase. It is more common among people over seventy years old. In the United States alone, more than sixty thousand cases of Parkinson's are diagnosed each year. Fifteen percent are individuals under the age of fifty.

Common Symptoms of Parkinson's Disease

- Tremors; shaking
- Rigidity; stiffness
- Freezing of gait
- Loss of taste
- Bradykinesia—moving very slowly
- Dementia
- Dystonia—abnormal muscle tone that can result in spasms or stooped posture
- Slow response to questions
- Blank facial expressions—poker face
- Short steps
- Micrographia—small, cramped handwriting
- Shuffling the feet
- Walking with the head down
- Anxiety
- Akinesia—inability to move
- Sniffling
- Crustiness around the eyes
- Uncharacteristically low and soft voice or slurred speech
- Seborrhea—flaky skin on the face and scalp
- Dysphasia—difficulty speaking or communicating
- Pain
- Loss of sexual appetite
- Depression
- Sleeplessness
- Urgency to urinate
- Loss of smell

The Five Stages of Parkinson's Disease

Stage 1   Tremors are on one side of the body. Symptoms are mild.

Stage 2   Symptoms become bilateral—both sides of the body are affected. Posture and gait are affected.

Stage 3   Very slow movement; walking and standing become difficult.

Stage 4   Symptoms become severe. Can only walk a short distance. Rigidity and movement are severe. Cannot live alone anymore.

Stage 5   Must use a wheelchair or remain in bed. Cannot stand or walk. Requires nursing care twenty-four hours a day.

Medications for Parkinson's Disease

Many medicines are used to treat this dreaded disease. Each one is used for different purposes. I myself take Mirapex and Sinemet. What works for me may not work for others. We are all different. Each individual's doctor will prescribe the right medicine. Never take medication prescribed for someone else. Always follow a doctor's advice.

Can You Die from Parkinson's Disease?

I've been told that you cannot die from Parkinson's disease. But, the truth is, you *can* die from Parkinson's.

Let me explain. When you are lying around doing nothing, you tend to gain weight; your muscles atrophy, and your heart must work harder because of your weight gain. Your bones tend to get more brittle, you worry a lot, and you usually eat more because you have nothing else to do while you watch television. This sedentary lifestyle can lead to coronary heart disease or, putting it mildly, heart failure.

That is why exercising is essential, and it should be a priority in your life. Exercise builds muscle, makes bones strong, and keeps your arteries clear so that blood carrying oxygen can flow freely and smoothly. Most of all, you will feel better. Remember: it's never too late to start.

When I first met Tom Gatses in 2003, I had the difficult task of telling him that although we might be able to improve his kidney function for a few more months, eventually he would need dialysis or kidney transplant to stay alive. Over the years, I have had to give this news to many people but Tom was different from any other patient I had seen. He had already struggled with Parkinson's disease for 4 years. Except for the mild tremor he had, I would never have known it. Far from having the mask like face sometimes described with Parkinson's, he was animated and filled with determination to fight the effects of both diseases. He maintained his health and high level of functioning with a grueling exercise regimen that would have made Arnold Schwarzenegger look like a slacker. He held off his kidney failure for 4 years. When he started dialysis, he chose to do home hemodialysis. This choice required bringing the type of machine usually used 3 times a week in dialysis centers to clean the blood into his home. Many patients are intimidated by the complex machine, but Tom saw it as a way to maintain his independence and take charge of his own health care. He continued his exercise program despite the fatigue that many people feel with dialysis. He mastered the use of the machine use and did his own dialysis until June of 2008 when a kidney transplant became available. His kidney has worked well but the years after transplant have not been smooth sailing. He required the removal of his old kidneys because of a suspicion of cancer. This required a bigger operation than the kidney transplant itself. The surgery left him temporarily weakened but he approached his recovery with the same determination that he has brought to every other medical problem he has faced. He has once again hit his stride and is providing inspiration and hope to other people with Parkinson's and with kidney failure. He has also provided an inspiration to his doctors and nurses who have come to recognize what a positive attitude and determination can do to make a difference in living with and overcoming serious illness.

Susan Hou

Why I Treat Parkinson's Disease as a Human Being

I treat Parkinson's not as a disease but as a human being. Because of my training in martial arts, I visualize myself fighting a man. This way, I feel as though I am defending myself against an enemy who deserves no mercy. I fear no one, especially Parkinson's. When "he" sees how good my support group is, he backs off. When he sees what a fantastic attitude I have, he keeps his distance. When Parkinson's sees how strong my faith is, he doesn't dare mess with me. And when he sees how much I exercise, he walks away in disgust and disappointment, hoping to try again the next day. As long as I am living my life the S.A.F.E. way, Parkinson's disease will never beat me.

My Experience with Parkinson's Disease

One day in early August 1999, I was driving my car, and my right hand was resting on my thigh. Suddenly, I noticed that my right index finger was twitching. I put it out of my mind, thinking it was just stress. A few days later, it happened again, and I thought, "I must really be stressed out!" For several weeks, the occasional twitching continued, but I figured it would eventually stop. My wife and I took a trip to Boston to visit our daughter, and, during dinner, my hand was shaking. Of course it was noticeable, and my wife grew very concerned. She also saw my arm shake occasionally. I told her I was just cold. But it just would not stop—and I could not control it.

My wife, Jennie, would not let it go. She sensed that something was seriously wrong. We went to our family doctor, and he said that he thought it was nothing serious; it was probably stress related. We went to a specialist, and he concurred with our family doctor—stress.

My wife did not feel comfortable with that diagnosis, so she researched doctors and specialists for Parkinson's disease. She just had the feeling there was something more to it than stress. She found Dr. Christopher Goetz through Rush Presbyterian St. Luke's Hospital in Chicago. I still refer to him as the best Parkinson's doctor there is.

Jennie made an appointment for me to see the doctor in early December of 1999.

As soon as Dr. Goetz examined me, he said that I had Parkinson's disease.

My heart sank, and I felt as though my life was about to go downhill. Immediately, I became depressed. My wife assured me that I was a strong man, and she reminded me that I could get through this. She tried to keep me from wallowing in self-pity and encouraged me to continue to exercise and take my mind off this weakening disease. She knew that I was making myself sicker by focusing on all the negative symptoms of this disease.

Everyone else seemed to feel sorry for me. I felt sorry for myself, too. Soon after that, my legs started tightening up. I was terrified that it would only be a matter of time before I wouldn't be able to walk. This would destroy me. I was never so scared in my life.

One day, I was lying on the couch feeling miserable, and my wife couldn't stand seeing me like that anymore. She firmly said, "Tom, what is wrong with you? You have four beautiful children, three of whom are boys, and they look up to you. Get up, and take control. You need to fight—for your kids! Why would you let your life end, and why would you want your kids to see you submit to this? They have always seen you as a fighter. My God; you're a fourth-degree black belt in karate and judo!"

At that moment, I decided that I was not going to let this disease take over my body and my mind. I was going to do whatever it took to control Parkinson's, not let Parkinson's control me. I started exercising again. This time I was exercising for my life. It was a different feeling, but let me tell you, it was a powerful feeling. I started working out in the water. I knew that water training was the best kind of training. I also rode my mountain bike several miles a day. I played racquetball once a week and tried to golf as much as I could. I did the stairs at Swallow Cliff—all 125 of them—and I thought I would have a heart attack, but I still did them. I walked often. Determination kept me going. Rather quickly, I felt myself getting stronger.

I visited Dr. Goetz three or four times a year, and each time he saw me, he said I was doing fine. Amazingly, I was still in the first stage of Parkinson's disease. I started feeling better and better about myself. I was keeping myself in the first stage. I was not going to allow Parkinson's disease to move any farther. I felt like I could write a book on my experiences with this disease. I continued to lift weights and exercise in the water. I seemed to be happiest when I was exercising.

I listened to my doctor and had plenty of support from my immediate family and closest friends. Most of all, I believed in myself again. I feel like I could stay like this the rest of my life. *If I can do this, anyone can,* I thought. I owe a lot to exercise, and I am very grateful that I had the encouragement I did from my wife and family. Of course, there were some who were in denial, and their confusion caused me more anxiety. They couldn't—or wouldn't—believe I had Parkinson's disease.

But through my wife's and children's support, I learned to ignore those comments and persevere through negative opinions.

I was also on the donor list for a kidney transplant. This was unrelated to Parkinson's disease, but it was another reason for me to feel down and depressed. But I decided that I just wouldn't give in. I own my body, and I will fight for it. I know that there are a lot of people who are worse off than I am, and I can only imagine what they must go through. I'm still working on playing the cards God dealt me, and I am going to play a good game.

Here I am, almost thirteen years later, and I am still in stage one. I am sixty-four years old, and I am still going strong. I just want to relay a message to anyone out there who has Parkinson's disease or any other debilitating ailment—and to every healthy individual out there as well—my advice is: Don't sit around and feel sorry for yourself. Live your life to its fullest. Start slow and gradually work yourself to a nice pace; exercise your self-pity away. You could be worse, and why give your disease a chance to progress? Use me as an example: *If Tom can do it, then I can do it!* Believe in yourself, and have faith. If you have family, get their support. Take it one day at a time. Listen to your doctor, take your medication, and exercise. My doctor is pleased with the way I am, and that means everything to me.

My Senses of Smell and Taste

Not long after I found out I had Parkinson's disease, my sense of smell disappeared. I couldn't smell anything. My doctor told me that I could eventually lose my sense of taste. I was very upset at the thought of never smelling again. I am Greek, and if you know anything about Greeks, they love to cook. The thought of never tasting my wife's cooking or smelling the scent of it when she makes dinner, was heartbreaking.

By some miracle, at my daughter's wedding, I smelled the incense in the church, *and* the red roses. Why red roses? I still do not know, but the smell brought tears to my eyes. I told my wife, and she squeezed my hand to let me know how happy she was for me. Soon after, I could start to smell different perfumes. I thought that maybe my sense of smell was returning.

I still don't know why I can smell some things, but let me tell you, the partial return of my sense of smell is one of those things that happened restored faith to my life. I prayed for months to be able to smell something, and finally, my prayers were answered. I think all the time that if I can smell again, that might mean that my disease is improving. I know that this is not the case, but when positive things happen and you have been praying for them, then little miracles seem like big miracles. I cling to these small miracles, and my faith carries me through each day in search of new ones. On a comical note, there are benefits of not smelling. For example; I cannot smell when my grandchildren's diapers need to be changed—that counts as a mini-miracle as well!

Choosing Your Doctor

When choosing your doctor, it is imperative to find the physician that is right for *you*. It is best to learn all you can about this person. After your first visit, you'll want to make sure that this is the right doctor for you; after all, there are many doctors in this field. Thanks to my wife and her research, we found Dr. Christopher Goetz.

Dr. Goetz is tops in his field at Rush Presbyterian St. Luke's Hospital in Chicago. He made me feel very comfortable, and he tells it like it is. He gives me regular checkups and keeps me informed on any new medicines for Parkinson's. His nurse, Lucy, is wonderful and is always there to answer any questions I have.

Getting a Second Opinion

You must always get a second and even a third opinion. You will feel better knowing that the doctors agree about your illness. If you are content with your doctor, stay there. Sometimes switching can be more harmful to your treatment. A new doctor may prescribe a new drug that could be harmful to you. As for myself, I feel very comfortable with Dr. Goetz. I wouldn't switch doctors if you paid me.

Some of my family and friends told me to go to the Mayo Clinic in Minnesota. Dr. Goetz assured me that if I wanted to go there, he would be more than happy to send me. The doctors at Mayo Clinic are Dr. Goetz's colleagues, and they would probably send me back to him. But I know that I am in good hands with Dr. Goetz.

Listen to Your Doctor

Meaning well, your relatives and friends will want to give you advice—but don't listen to them about your disease. Many of them will offer their opinions on what to do and which medicines to take. Some of them are also in denial, because they don't want to believe that you have Parkinson's disease.

Some of my friends and relatives give me articles or tell me about new drugs that are out. I just tell all these people that if my doctor wants me to take other drugs he will tell me so. People don't understand. If I switch medicines, it could be detrimental to my health. In my case, being in the first stage and doing exceptionally well, I don't have to feel as if I should have to take other drugs.

So, while people mean well, they are ignorant in this field. They will give their opinions, suggest that you don't have Parkinson's, that you have a nervous condition or some other problem.

My doctor advised me that if all my friends and relatives are constantly recommending for me to try something new or telling me that I shouldn't be exercising so much, I should tell them to please contact him. He can tell them in person not to interfere. They may be well-meaning, but they don't realize the damage they could cause me by disrupting my regimen. The old adage, "Too many cooks spoil the soup" is something to keep in mind.

My Family Doctor

Perhaps one of the most important people in my life is my family physician, Dr. Robert Sulo. He is, in my opinion, the greatest general practitioner at both Loyola and Palos hospitals. I have never seen a more dedicated doctor. He is at one of the hospitals as early as 4:30 a.m., making his rounds. He travels to both hospitals and then goes to his clinic. How he does this is beyond my imagination. On top of a long day at the clinic, he makes his phone calls, usually after 9:00 p.m., to his patients to discuss their lab work. Not only is he a caring doctor, he is a fantastic doctor as well.

I consider it an honor to know such a wonderful human being. Dr. Sulo is always there for me, and I always listen to his advice. God bless you Dr. Sulo. You will always be in my prayers. Thank you for everything.

Psychology and Parkinson's

When I first met with Dr. Bernard, a psychologist, at Rush Medical Center in Chicago, I was very nervous. I didn't know what to expect. But Dr. Bernard made me feel very comfortable and calm. His job was to test my memory and help me cope with my disease. He has been a big help to me and has concluded that my memory is very good.

Always keep your mind occupied and work on your memory. This will help you to keep your sanity. Talk to a psychologist and tell him your problems and what bothers you. He is there to help you, not hurt you.

Incidentally, I can name every country and capital in the world. My memory hasn't been affected by Parkinson's. I keep my mind busy by doing puzzles and reading a lot of educational material. I am grateful to Dr. Bernard for his assistance, and I will continue to visit him regularly.

SS CONSTANTINE AND HELEN GREEK ORTHODOX CHURCH

11025 South Roberts Road *(Honorary Fr. Byron Way)* • Palos Hills, Illinois 60465

708.974.3400 • Fax 708.974.0179

www.stconstantinehelen.org

Mr. Tom Gatses
16120 Georgetown Sq.
Orland Park, IL 60467

April 19, 2011

My Very Dear Friend and Co-Struggler, Tom;

Christ is Risen – Truly He is Risen! With the joy of the Resurrection of our Lord and Saviour Jesus Christ, I write you and commend you on this your present work.

In my salutation above, I addressed you as "co-struggler". We all struggle together through this life, yet you my dear friend, have moved the bar to an all time high. You, dear Tom, as I have told you many times, are an example for others. You are an inspiration for me personally. I feel unworthy to be in the same class as you, because you have allowed God to pick you up to heights I do not think I can ever reach.

I am always overwhelmed with people like you, who take the heavy Cross of their life and carry it not grudgingly…but joyfully…allowing it to be used as a "bridge" that will carry them over the canyons of life.

I thank God for allowing our paths of cross. My life is all the more blessed because of you!

Fr. Nicholas W. Jonas
Pastor

Father Nicholas W. Jonas, *Pastor*   Father Byron Papanikolaou, *Protopresbyter*   Father Tom DeMedeiros, *Presbyter*

Mr. John Arvanetes, *Parish Council President*   Mr. Theodore P. Argiris, *Chairman of the Board*

Depression and Parkinson's

Being depressed will not help you with any illness. We all experience depression at one time or another and in different degrees. Talking to someone about it and educating yourself can be more of a help than you can imagine. There is always someone to talk to, whether it is a counselor, your family, your nurse, your doctor, a friend, or even a stranger. You need to build your confidence and self-esteem and slowly build yourself back up so you can fight your illness.

I went through depression when I first found out I had Parkinson's disease. I just wanted to be left alone. Through the support and encouragement of my family, I stopped feeling sorry for myself and started to fight this disease. My family reminded me that I had never been beaten before, so why should I go down without a fight now?

Also, I started praying. I started talking about my feelings. I started exercising and utilizing all my resources. I started developing my idea for S.A.F.E living, and my depression seemed to disappear. Now, don't get me wrong, there are many times I can fall right back into feeling sorry for myself. But I firmly remind myself that I will fail this if I don't keep going. I will not succumb to this disease easily. I will fight it off the best way I know how, and that is the S.A.F.E way.

Stress and Parkinson's

Being stressed out will push your disease to the next stage if you let it. Don't listen to anyone except your doctor about your disease; they don't know your history. Don't let your bills or other stressors take over your sanity. We all have bills, and we all have problems. Even the rich have problems, some of them more than others. Just live your life one day at a time, and try not to worry. I know it is difficult when you fall behind on your bills, but, believe me, worrying constantly about money or health or whatever else bothers you will just make your disease progress.

Listen to your doctor and do as he says. Think positive thoughts, and don't let anything or anyone get you down. You must take charge of your own self and have a positive attitude.

Exercise and Parkinson's

When my doctor told me that it was imperative that I exercise at least one hour a day, I felt good. I have been exercising all my life, sometimes many hours a day.

Remember, with Parkinson's, your muscles start to stiffen up, especially in your legs. But exercise will make you feel better and keep you going. Without exercising, you will progress more rapidly. With regular exercise, your Parkinson's will slow down, and you will feel better. Almost any exercise can be helpful, but it is up to you. Either exercise and fight this dreaded disease—or sit around and let it overtake you. You are exercising for your life. If need be, get a personal trainer.

I am my own trainer. With my background and history of exercising and my will to work out, I found that the best way to fight Parkinson's is to remain active and ask for help.

There are many people on your side who will help you. Don't be a fool and sit around worrying about your disease. Do something about it—and live a healthier life. Look at me; many people can't believe I have Parkinson's, especially after twelve years. Just remember that you have the power and will to do it yourself. Either do it or suffer the consequences. No one will force you. You must make your own decision.

Choosing the Right Exercise

You may choose from many types of exercise and activities, but first, you must have the will to do it. Next, you must enjoy what you are doing. This will make exercise more fun. If you can't exercise on your own, ask for help. Sometimes when you are with someone else, you feel like competing, which can make you do more and get you going.

I myself have found that exercising regularly has been a key to keeping my Parkinson's from progressing any further. I have the right formula and am happy to share it with others. Keep your body active, and your life with Parkinson's—or any other disease—will be much easier. I can't tell you which exercises will work for you. I know is that exercise will help you, though, no matter what form you choose. Just do it.

Hydrotherapy

Water is, by far, the best place to exercise. I will argue that with anyone. The resistance you get will strengthen your muscles much faster, with less risk of injury, than other ways of working out. Swimming will help you use every muscle in your body. But, as with all exercise, even in the water, you must listen to your body. If it feels like you are doing too much, lighten up. Remember, Rome wasn't built in a day. It takes time to build up endurance, and only you can make it happen.

There are many exercises you can do in the water. Use intervals of five minutes. First walk forward, then walk backward. Next, walk sideways, first to your right and then to your left, again in five minute intervals. Then, alternate lifting your legs up until your knee touches your chest or comes close, and repeat, alternating legs, for five minutes. For the next five minutes, concentrate on working your arms by swinging them back and forth. After working your arms, do twists from side to side by rotating your abdomen for five minutes, then add downward punches for another five-minute set. Then, finish by swimming laps for about five minutes. In forty-five minutes, you will have worked almost every muscle in your body.

Soon you will start to feel better and better, and this exercise will become routine in about two weeks. Do these workouts at least five days a week. The results will amaze you.

Weight Lifting

In Parkinson's, your muscles tend to tighten up quickly. Working out with weights will help build your muscles so you can regain the strength you have lost. Start off with light weights, and do several repetitions. Remember to start gradually. You may feel like you are wasting your time, but, believe me, weights will help. In no time at all, you will feel stronger. You can gradually increase the weight as time goes by. For those of you who say, "I can't do it,"—that is unacceptable. Just try; push yourself. Remember, you are not like you used to be. Get a personal trainer if you must. Just do it, and the results will speak for themselves.

No matter what illness you have, if you don't exercise, your bones will become weak, and your muscles will atrophy. That is why working out with weights is imperative. You don't need heavy weights. Light weights, with several repetitions, will suffice. I don't recommend free weights because they are harder to control. Nautical machines are much safer. There are about 640 muscles in the human body. Whatever exercise or activity you engage in, you will be using different muscle groups.

I recommend the following workout, which is especially great for people with Parkinson's:

- Leg Press—great for strengthening both upper and lower leg muscles
- Arm Curls—for biceps and forearms
- Bench Press—for chest and arms
- Crunches—for abs
- Triceps Extensions—for arms, chest, and triceps

There are many machines you can use. Try a variety of machines, and select which ones work best for you. Ask a trainer to show you how to use them properly so that you can avoid accidental injury. The best time to work out is whenever you have time. Mornings are preferred by many because, after a good workout and a nice shower, you will feel great the rest of the day.

Resistance Bands

The best type of resistance band is the ones that have hand grips. There are five exercises that I do—and recommend that you do—at least five days per week. You'll need a chair and some type of immovable post to wrap the bands around. These exercises are fantastic for building up and strengthening your upper body, including your arms, chest, shoulders, and back.

Exercise 1—Sit in a chair facing the post, about four or five feet away from the post. Wrap the bands around the pole and grip firmly with palms turned inward. Now, pull slowly toward your chest and release slowly back to original position; repeat twenty-five times.

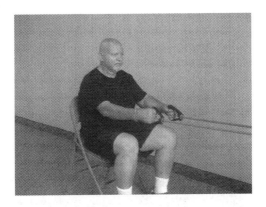

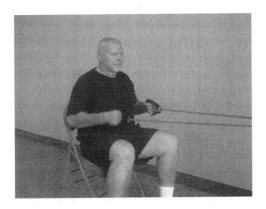

* Muscles involved: chest and back

Exercise 2—Turn your chair around away from the post and put it about one foot away. As bands are wrapped around the pole, grip them on each side with your palms inward. Now push them outward, slowly extending your arms and retracting back to your starting position. Do twenty-five repetitions.

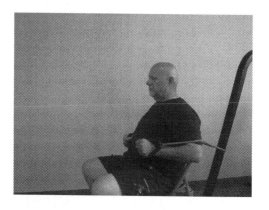

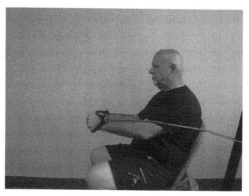

* Muscles involved: back, arms, chest

Exercise 3—Stand up, facing any direction; with both feet on the center of the band, grasp each end of the band with your hands. With your feet no more than shoulder width apart, shrug your shoulders upward and then relax. Repeat this twenty-five times.

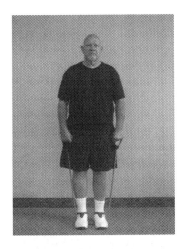 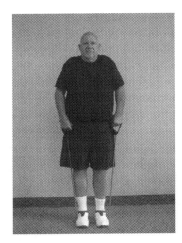

* Muscles involved: shoulders and trapezius

Exercise 4—Stand facing the post, with the band wrapped around the post; grasp ends with both hands waist high. With your arms slightly bent and palms facing back, pull the band back as far as you can, hold for a second, and go back to your original position. Repeat twenty-five times.

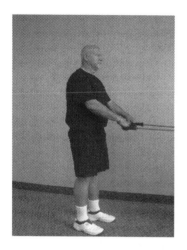 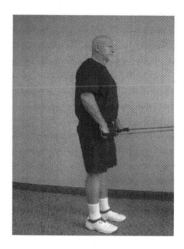

* Muscles involved: triceps and forearms

Exercise 5—Place chair facing post, about four or five feet away. While in a sitting position, wrap band around the post and grasp each end with both hands, with palms facing up. With your arms slightly bent and elbows at your sides, pull or curl the band upward, toward your shoulders, then go back to your original position. Repeat twenty-five times.

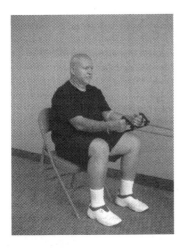 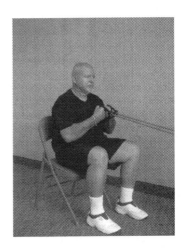

* Muscles involved: biceps and forearms

When these exercises start to become less difficult, you can add another band or increase the number of repetitions that you do. I use two bands and do these exercises one hundred times each. Every time I do these exercises, I feel stronger and look more muscular. The results will inspire you to keep going.

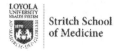

Loyola University Chicago
Stritch School of Medicine

Department of Neurological Surgery
Tel: (708) 216-3208
Fax: (708) 216-4948

March 8, 2011

Having known Tom Gatses for a number of years, in a relationship which is both clinical and personal, I can attest to the fact that this is one remarkable individual. Tom has not let the ravages of Parkinson's disease dampen his personal or religious beliefs or his family life.

This patient has taught me a lot about how an individual wages war against this devastating disease. There is no doubt that his physical exercise program keeps him in wonderful shape. His family relationships knit that unit together. His wonderful wife gives him the encouragement he needs to get through each day.

Tom Gatses has taught me how to wage the war, how keeping physically and emotionally strong helps one get through each day. This involves maximum effort; however, its rewards make the effort seem trivial because of what is gained. Two hours of exercise each day keeps you ten steps in front of the ravages of this disease.

I congratulate Tom on his new edition.

Thank you.

John F. Shea, MD

John F. Shea, M.D.
Professor, Neurological Surgery

Bicycling

Remember, with Parkinson's, your legs start to get rigid. You might start to feel as if you can't walk anymore. Get on a life cycle, and start to pedal. When you feel your legs getting a little stronger—which they will—buy yourself a mountain bike.

I ride my bike as much as I can. My legs feel stronger, and it motivates me to do more. I ride for miles. I don't fall asleep because I am constantly moving.

On a bicycle, you will feel much more alert because you are on two wheels and you don't want to crash. Bicycling is an excellent way to build muscles and gain strength in your legs. For many people with Parkinson's, it won't be easy, so start off by going around the block. The next day, ride around two blocks. Before you know it, you will be riding many miles. You will enjoy riding more as time goes by. A mountain bike is best because you can ride off road as well as on the road.

Walking

Walking provides excellent exercise, not only for Parkinson's but for your heart as well. Start off walking slowly, and build yourself up to a brisk walk. Walk around the block, and, every day go a little bit farther until you get to at least half an hour a day of walking. Walk with good posture, and your whole body will benefit from the exercise. Walking uses many different muscles, and you will soon see improvement in your strength. While walking, twist your body now and then and move your arms up and down. There are many things you can do while walking. Don't just say you're going to do it—do it, and you will feel the difference. Wear a good pair of gym shoes that provide support and, most of all, comfort.

Flexibility

Always stretch to warm up before participating in any exercise or activity. This will improve your performance and reduce the chance of injury. If you need assistance stretching, get a partner to help you. The more you stretch, the better your chances of preventing injury to your body. Remember to start gradually and keep working slowly, until you are able to do it alone and you feel more confident. I always say it's never too late. Stretch, and you will see the difference.

Exercising while Lying Down

Some exercises can be done when you are lying on your back. Lift one leg up and then lower it. Now do the same with the other leg. If you can, lift both legs up at the same time and then lower them. Holding them up for a while will increase your strength. Next, bring your leg to your chest, using your hands to pull it toward you. Then lower your leg. Now do the same with the other leg. After that, bring both legs up to your chest. Then lower them.

Now, work on your arms. Raise them over your head then bring them down. Next lift your arms to your sides at shoulder height. Then lower them.

Raise your head, then lay it back down. Now turn your head to one side, then the other.

To increase your strength, hold all of these positions for a few seconds or longer.

Exercising from a Wheelchair

For those of you who use a wheelchair and, because of that, think that you cannot exercise, remember—if you can move any part of your body, then you can exercise. Take, for example, a can of peas, soup, or corn. Grasp the can in your hand and raise it over your head, then lower your arm. Next, throw punches, still holding the can.

To work the muscles in your legs, lift each left leg and lower it. Next, kick your legs out and bring them back—one at a time or both at the same time.

Next, try to touch your chin to your chest. Then tilt your head back. After that, turn your head to one side, then the other.

Exercises I Do and Recommend

First of all, I enjoy exercise. I have been doing it all my life. I am doing so well with my Parkinson's because I exercise every day. It is imperative that people with Parkinson's disease—or any other disease—exercise at least five days per week. Exercise is the key to fighting Parkinson's or any other disease you may have. You will feel better, and you will be able to function much more easily.

I lift weights, swim, bicycle, practice martial arts, play racquetball, and golf. I also exercise my mind by playing chess, backgammon, and Scrabble and by doing crossword puzzles. I have also memorized the names of countries of the world and their capitals. I will not allow Parkinson's disease to stop me from enjoying all of these things and more.

The Effects of Not Exercising for Extended Lengths of Time

When I was told by my doctor to exercise daily, I was very happy. When I had surgery for my kidneys, I was not allowed to exercise for a few months. In no time at all, I felt like my body started to fall apart.

I started aching and my legs became more rigid. Putting my socks on became more and more difficult. It became hard to bend down. It felt like my disease was progressing.

I couldn't wait to work out again. When I was cleared to resume activity, it didn't take me long to start feeling better. I quickly jumped back into my routine and regained my strength. Remember, I am a fighter, and I can't—rather, I will not—yield to Parkinson's disease or to any other illness. As long as I live the S.A.F.E way, I believe that I can overcome anything.

How I Slow Down the Progression of My Parkinson's Disease

We all know that there is no cure for Parkinson's disease. Those of us who have it, unfortunately, must learn to live with it. Be strong and thankful that you don't have cancer, MS, or something else that is worse than Parkinson's. I, for one, said, "Why me, God? All my life I exercised and got involved in many activities. What did I do to deserve this?" I thought that maybe God was testing me and helping me cope with this disease until a cure is available.

As for me, I won't let this disease destroy my life. I have support from family, relatives, and friends. But if you give up and don't do anything about it, then don't expect to last long.

To stay ahead of Parkinson's, you must have a positive attitude and keep active. Exercise is the best way to fight this incurable disease. When you exercise, your muscles get stronger. Your blood flows more freely throughout your body, carrying the oxygen that you need. Your organs, especially your heart, benefit from your exercise.

Remember, the hardest muscle to build up is your heart. A person who is in good shape has fewer heartbeats per minute and better blood flow throughout his body. Exercising helps you build strong bones and muscles.

I recommend that you target an area where you are weak and strengthen that part of your body. For example; if your legs are weak and stiff, you must concentrate on building muscle and strength in these limbs. My legs started to stiffen up first, so I worked on them until I felt normal again. It won't take long for you to build up your strength in your whole body. Just have faith and the will to survive. Look at people with worse diseases; they might wish that they had the opportunity to do something about their problems. They can't, but you can, and you must. Don't feel sorry for yourself; just say, *I have the disease and I accept it and I must do something to fight it.* Either you will do this or you will suffer the consequences.

The Effects Other Medicines Have on My Parkinson's Disease

Parkinson's disease has had a devastating impact on my entire family, although I am the one who must take medication to control my condition. The medications help tremendously, but at a price. For one thing, they lower my blood pressure, which causes me to get lightheaded when I bend down to pick something up or when I try to put my shoes on. I also get extremely tired throughout the day. I might just close my eyes, and next thing I know, I am dreaming. I stopped driving for a few years because of this.

Another effect of the medicine is that I have a lot of anxiety. I am always in a hurry, and when I want something done, I have to do it right away. A good example is this book. Although it has taken some time to put my thoughts into words, my anxiety over completing it has caused major conflicts with my family members. I kept nagging my children to help me on the computer, to type, and to help me edit. I showed no concern about them, the fact that they have other things to do during the day; with my anxiety, I feel like "it is all about me." I know that they are all married with children and other responsibilities, but I just wanted my book to be completed.

My anxiety caused a lot of unnecessary grief, and, even though they have supported me through this endeavor, it has been a difficult path because of both my Parkinson's disease and the side effects of my medication.

The last major side effect I have is I that I have very vivid dreams. This can be comical, yet it can also be dangerous. One time, while my wife was driving, I fell asleep. Now, I am a black belt in karate and I have learned how to break bricks with my hands. So, my wife was driving and I fell asleep, and I started dreaming about breaking a brick. Well my wife tells me that stared, in awe, at what I was doing. My right arm went up in the air, and, suddenly, I yelled as I do in karate, and my hand came down, striking my left thigh with a karate chop. Of course, I woke up from the intense pain, and a huge bruise developed from the impact. But my wife was certainly scared! What if I dreamed of fighting with someone else, and I attacked my wife? The vivid dreams are a serious side effect of the medication.

On top of the Parkinson's disease and all the side effects of my medication, I also had renal deficiency. My kidneys were working only at about 10 percent of normal function, and they were failing more and more each day. Because of my poor kidney function, the medicines I took were not being filtered through my kidneys fast enough; it was taking about four times as long as it should have for my kidneys to filter the medicines. Therefore, a lot of my side effects were the result of my body acting like I had "overdosed." This altered my moods as well as my personality, increasing my agitation. Every little thing bothered me. With heightened anxiety, I became very argumentative with my family. Imagine what my family must have gone through because of my ailments and the side effects of my medication!

Another side effect of medication for Parkinson's disease is addiction. You might have read about a correlation between Parkinson's disease and gambling. Well, for me this was true. I have always enjoyed playing cards and the occasional casino trip, as most people would. Now, however, it seemed to be an obsession. There were times that I spent my entire disability check at the casino boat. I was always trying to find money and looking for ways to buy scratch tickets. Not even the dollar tickets seemed to be good enough—I needed to buy the ten- and twenty-dollar tickets. I seemed to be always searching for a big payoff, even though the odds were against me. It seems that the medication altered my ability to behave rationally.

Of course, when you gamble, the chances of winning are slim, so I would lose what I had, then lack the money to pay our bills, a cycle that created additional anxiety. It became a vicious cycle.

On a recent visit to my doctor, my wife told him of my behavior. Dr. Goetz explained that it wasn't my fault—it was due to the medicine I take and its effect on my emotions. He explained that, because it was taking so long for my kidneys to filter out my medicine, the effect was that I felt like an alcoholic, gambler, or drug addict. Dr. Goetz did cut down on my medication and since, it has helped but there are still episodes. Because of the lower dose of medicine, my tremors have increased a bit. Dr. Goetz was concerned with how this would affect me, but I have assured him that I would rather have slight tremors than create havoc in our home with the side effects of the higher dose. I can still play racquetball, ride my bike, swim, and work out with weights. And, as long as I am able to maintain my S.A.F.E way of living, everything else seems to fall into place.

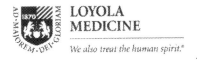

January 4, 2011

To Whom It May Concern:

I met Tom Gatses in June, 2008 when I became his post-renal transplant coordinator, shortly after he received a kidney transplant from a deceased donor after waiting four years on the transplant waiting list. Tom had been on hemodialysis to clean his blood for two years before he received the kidney transplant. I learned that he was also afflicted with Parkinson's Disease, which caused him to have tremors and affected his ability to walk normally.

Despite Tom's medical problems, he has always maintained a positive and energetic attitude and refuses to allow his illnesses take over his life. In 2009 he was rehospitalized for major abdominal surgery to repair a hernia and had several setbacks following this surgery. His recovery was delayed due to the extent of the surgery and related complications, however he ultimately prevailed, returning to daily intense workouts at the gym. Since I have known Tom, exercise has always been an important part of his life and probably one of the reasons he is able to bounce back from illness to health successfully.

In addition to his cheerful attitude and determination to stay fit with regular exercise, Tom also participates in the care of his grandchildren, some being toddlers in the "terrible 2s". This is no easy job for even the healthiest adult, but Tom does it with joy and enthusiasm and cherishes the time he spends with his extended family.

I am grateful that I have a profession that allows me to interact with inspirational people like Tom. Knowing him gives me courage that I too, may be able to overcome the ravages of a serious illness or other devastating event that could occur in my own life someday. Tom has taught me that it pays off to never give up or let adverse events destroy one's spirit.

Sincerely,

Anita L. Pakrasi, R.N.
Renal Transplant Coordinator
Loyola University Medical Center

Surgery and Parkinson's

Surgery is performed as a last resort for some Parkinson's patients, but so far it has not been successful in curing these patients of this debilitating disease. Before considering surgery, make sure that you have tried all other avenues. I do not advise undertaking a surgical procedure unless your doctor deems it necessary for you. If all other avenues have proven unsuccessful and your doctor feels that there is hope with surgery, then by all means go for it. If this can slow down the progression of Parkinson's and ease your pain for a little while, it may be worth the risk.

Support Groups

Support groups offer help for those who have Parkinson's disease. It is often helpful to meet with others who can relate to the problems you are having because they have the same illness and have had similar experiences. Many people with Parkinson's are afraid to attend a support group because they do not think it will help. But you won't know until you go to the meeting. We must support each other. Is it in these groups that we can realize that we are *not* alone. You can then talk about your disease because everyone in the group shares the pain. Get it out. Don't hold anything in. The people in a support group can help you get through your bad times. We must support each other.

Talking to People about Parkinson's Disease

Since I am doing so well, I thought, *why not share my secret on how I am slowing the process of Parkinson's disease progression?* Speaking to an audience and helping motivate even one person would make me feel that I am changing myself as well. I wish that all patients of Parkinson's and other ailments lived by the same philosophy. Depression might not become such huge factor if people felt less alone, and the physical well-being of many people could improve. People might say that talk is cheap. This may very well be, but I honestly practice what I preach. Encouraging just one person makes the effort worthwhile.

The Benefits of Having a Positive Attitude

Having a positive attitude is a good way to increase dopamine in your brain, says Dr. Christopher Goetz of Rush Presbyterian St. Luke's Hospital in Chicago, Illinois. Low levels of dopamine cause the symptoms of Parkinson's disease.

In addition to increasing dopamine, having a positive attitude will change your perception of your illness. I have a positive attitude because I use one word—S.A.F.E.—in my everyday living. Think positive and witness the results. I made my choice, Now, it's up to *you*!!

Do I Have Parkinson's Disease or
Does Parkinson's Disease Have Me?

I use reverse psychology on this disease. It may sound crazy to most people, but it works for me. Why should I have Parkinson's? Why shouldn't Parkinson's disease have me? When I look at things this way, Parkinson's disease is fighting me. I enjoy meeting Parkinson's disease on a daily basis. "He" never knows when I will strike or what is going on inside my mind. All he is concerned about is getting rid of me. I know that Parkinson's disease is confused and disoriented knowing that I invaded his body. This is one of the reasons I am doing so well. Let Parkinson's disease worry about me and my positive attitude instead of me worrying about him.

Laughing at Parkinson's

Laughter is a wonderful way of promoting wellness. Laughing at your disease may improve your health. Some people say that laughter is a good way to fight your illness—any illness. When you laugh at Parkinson's disease or any other sickness, it's very possible that your progression could slow down. Those of us who have a good sense of humor have an open mind. Others may see laughter as offensive and avoid discussing their illnesses. I laugh at my disease, and I make jokes about it all the time. This shows that I am winning. On the other hand, crying means that Parkinson's is winning. Think about it; would you laugh and be happy or would you cry and be sad? Don't give in to Parkinson's or any other illness. Laugh, and live your life to its fullest.

Walking with Your Head Down

When you walk with your head down, Parkinson's is controlling you. When you look down, you are looking at the devil. Parkinson's disease knows he has you—and he is laughing his head off. Look up, anywhere above ground, and face God. This will upset Parkinson's disease, and he will back off. Slowly your posture will get better as time goes by. Walk proudly, and keep that positive attitude working. After all, who is in command of your body, you or Parkinson's disease? Fight and don't ever stop fighting. You only fail when you give up.

Shuffling or Taking Short Steps

When you walk with short steps or you shuffle your feet, Parkinson's has you.

By taking longer steps and lifting your feet a little higher, you will leave Parkinson's disease behind you.

The more you walk with longer strides, the farther back you will leave Parkinson's. And when you do walk, pretend that you are walking on him. Don't be lenient. He doesn't care about you, so don't worry about him. Now that you are ahead, don't let Parkinson's disease catch you. Even though it might be difficult, try your best. Just try to walk like a normal person. Be proud of yourself, and take care of your body. I know it will not be easy, but if you keep a positive attitude, soon you will see and feel the difference.

What Puzzles Me Most about
My Parkinson's Disease

I have had Parkinson's for more than twelve and a half years. I am happy to say that I am still in my first stage. I feel better now than I ever did. I exercise daily. I have one of the best attitudes in the world, and I belong to one of the best support groups anyone could ever ask for. My faith is unbelievable, and I take my medicines every day. After all the beatings Parkinson's disease gets from me, you would think he would leave me alone. But as stubborn as he is, I am just as stubborn. In the long run, only one of us will emerge victorious. I pity Parkinson's.

Sleeping with Parkinson's

Sleep disturbances are a common problem for people with Parkinson's. Let your doctor know that you have trouble sleeping so he can help correct this problem. Why torment yourself? There are many people with sleep disorders—hallucinations, violent dreams, and restless leg syndrome. So many Parkinson's disease patients can't wait to fall asleep. Some of our symptoms subside when we fall asleep. There are medicines that may help you to sleep better. Exercising will definitely help because working out makes you tired.

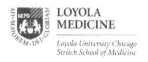

January 11, 2011

Mr. Tom Gatses
14317 S. Pebble Creek Drive
Homer Glen, IL 60491

To Whom It May Concern:

I have had the pleasure of knowing Tom for several years now, as one of his treating physicians. He is an extraordinarily positive individual who has battled life threatening medical conditions, rallying against adversity on a number of occasions. He is well aware of the power of a positive attitude in healing, and his jovial spirit has served him well in this regard. I am happy to know that he is sharing his experience and approach with others.

As a transplant surgeon who deals with life and death on a daily basis, I am a believer in the power of the spirit in healing, and agree with Tom that a healthy spirit and positive attitude are essential when one is facing a life threatening medical diagnosis. The recovery process is most certainly affected by one's mind-set. On a more profound note, I believe a positive outlook is essential no matter what medical outcome is rendered for each and every one of us.

Sincerely,

John E. Milner, M.D.
Transplant Surgeon
Loyola University, Chicago

MRSA and My Parkinson's

I had never heard of MRSA until I got my first attack. I was sitting in the kitchen shaking and freezing. I thought I was coming down with the flu. I didn't know that I could lose my life because of this deadly infection. If my wife hadn't called 911, I probably would have died.

I was taken to the hospital emergency room. The nurse took my temperature, which was almost 106. The doctor immediately admitted me. I was immediately given a room; when you have MRSA, you are automatically put in a room by yourself so you won't spread it to anyone else.

In eight months, I had MRSA infections five times. The last time was the worst. A fistula is an enlarged vein created by connecting an artery directly to a vein. This creates a much greater blood flow into the vein making inserting needles for hemodialysis treatments easier. My fistula got infected, leaving a bubble the size of a golf ball on my left arm. My doctor called for a vascular specialist, Dr. Dean Govostis, who is tops in his field. When he looked at my infection, he said that if it popped, I would not survive. In no time, I was on the operating table.

After it was over, my doctor told me that, because of my attitude and faith, I had pulled through. He said that the average man would never make it with all the infections I had. But after reading my book, he said, "now I know why you made it with all the MRSA infections you had; you are a fighter." I told him that I certainly am.

It's War!

Parkinson's disease deliberately entered my body in hopes of destroying me. As far as I'm concerned, this is an act of war. It has been, so far, a twelve-year battle. I seem to be winning, but Parkinson's disease is very sneaky. He could strike again at any time, affecting any part of my body. I don't use guns, tanks, grenades, or weapons of mass destruction. I use all the resources I have at hand, though. I use the S.A.F.E. method to combat this terrible disease. I enjoy a good fight; don't you?

My Dialysis

When it was time for me to go on dialysis, I prepared myself by keeping a positive attitude. I did not know what to expect.

When the nurse injected my arm for the first time, I could not believe how thick the needle was. Did it hurt? Indeed it did. She injected me several times and could not hit my fistula, the access point where the blood travels to the dialysis machine. The fistula moved every time the needle came near it. Two other nurses tried to insert the needle. After the nurses had made several attempts, my wife saw that I was in tremendous pain. She told the nurses to stop.

"Can't you people see how much pain my husband is in?" she demanded.

The nurses stopped and told us to go back to the doctor and have him redo the operation, fixing the fistula so that it wouldn't move. My doctor said that nothing was wrong with my fistula. But at the suggestion of my wife, the doctor repeated the surgery.

The next time my wife and I went to the dialysis center, I was ready to be dialyzed. I could not believe how much was involved in the process. There were so many steps to go through.

Once, during training, the nurse took too much fluid from my body and I passed out. After the nurse woke me up, my wife asked, "what if my husband passes out and no one is around to wake him up?"

The nurse said, "He would most likely die."

When I was being dialyzed at home, it took anywhere from two to three hours, five days a week. After each session, I felt a surge of energy going through my body. It was a nice feeling, and not what I had expected; I heard that, after being dialyzed, I would be very weak and tired the rest of the day.

After a year and a half of dialysis, I finally got a kidney transplant. The operation took about three and a half hours. My new kidney worked immediately. So here I am—stronger, older, and ready to take on the world. At sixty-four years of age, I consider myself to be in excellent condition. Having a positive attitude definitely helped.

Why Dialysis Did Not Affect
My Parkinson's Disease

Dialysis is the process of cleansing the blood of impurities. Most, if not all, medicines taken within a few hours before being dialyzed will be filtered out during the dialysis. This will most likely have an impact on your body. The best way to keep medicines from being discarded is to take them after dialysis. This way, your medications will be absorbed by your body before your next treatment.

Most people become very weak and tired for several hours after being dialyzed. But I always became energized after my treatments. One reason for that is that my dialysis was done five days per week. And it was done at home: *Home Hemo Dialysis.* My daughter, Christine, and my son Tommy took training to learn how to administer dialysis. Having dialysis at home improved my quality of life significantly. I felt bad for my children because they sacrificed their family time just to help me. But they wouldn't have it any other way. Thank God we are a close family

Medicines I Take for My New Kidney

Since my kidney transplant, I have had to take several different kinds of medicine. Some of the pills cause me to gain weight, while others cause me to become tired and weak. I thought that this would cause my Parkinson's to progress to the next level, but I was lucky. I am still in my first stage. I will be taking medicines for the rest of my life. But this does not bother me at all; it sure beats going back on dialysis.

Surgeries Not Related to Parkinson's

It is possible that surgeries and other procedures could affect your Parkinson's disease. I have had about fifty procedures and surgeries over the last five years, so I prepared myself for any result. I prayed that my Parkinson's disease would not progress. I was very lucky. You have to remember that I am a fighter. And fighters with a positive attitude always win.

The Caretaker

Do you have a chronic illness? If you think you have a rough time, look at your caretakers. Your caretaker not only has to cope with everyday living but with your illness as well.

Caretaking is like fighting a battle; it can drain your caretaker to complete exhaustion. The caretaker has the responsibility of driving you to the doctor, to the stores, or wherever else you need to go. Your caretaker must prepare your meals, bathe you, do your laundry, and do all of the other chores that you are unable to perform. As your disease progresses, it becomes more difficult for your caretaker as well. It's almost like taking care of a child—only much more difficult. Helping you get in and out of the car or a wheelchair, or even getting you in and out of the bed is more challenging because you are so much heavier than a child.

My wife is my caretaker. She has done so much for me, and I cannot thank her enough. Thank God, I work my program and try to stay ahead of my disease. It not only makes it easier on my wife but on my entire family. I can only imagine how other caretakers deal with their spouses. The next time you feel like complaining about yourself, think of your caretaker. At least someone is there for you. Who is there for your caretaker?

Parkinson's Deserves Pain and Suffering

Parkinson's entered my body with the intent of doing harm not only to me, but to my family as well. Because when I suffer, everyone else suffers. Parkinson's, you made a big and fatal mistake when you entered my body. Through my S.A.F.E. method, I am going to show you what pain and suffering really is. You can't escape because I won't let you. With my support group, *you* will hurt. With my positive attitude, you will cringe. With my faith, you will become disoriented, and with my exercising, you will scream in agony—and no one will hear you. This will go on until a cure is found. So suffer, you scum bag!

Dr. Susan Hou

When I first met Dr. Hou, I knew I had one of the best nephrologists at Loyola Hospital. I could see how much she cared for her patients. And I saw how impressed she was with the way I exercised.

Dr. Hou thought I would be on dialysis very soon, so she put me on the transplant list immediately. I am forever grateful to Dr. Hou, because it took another two years before I had to start dialysis.

I will never forget the time that Dr. Hou said I was an inspiration to everyone. After I had my kidney transplant operation, Dr. Hou was one of the first people I saw when I woke in recovery. It was like seeing an angel over my bed. I hugged and kissed her.

God bless you, Dr. Hou, and thank you for everything.

Dr. Demetrius Zikos

This wonderful doctor made it possible for me to have dialysis taken at my home. Every time I visited Dr. Zikos with my wife, he made me feel very relaxed and comfortable. He said that, because of my attitude, I was qualified to be dialyzed at home five or six days a week. That might sound like a lot, but it is not. It was far less time than the three days a week at the dialysis center would have taken.

Any time we needed to ask the doctor questions, he was there for us. I had MRSA five times in eight months, and Dr. Zikos told me that the average man would probably have died. But after reading my book, he said, "Now I know why you made it all the times you had MRSA. You are a fighter."

I will never forget you, Dr. Zikos. Thank you for all your help and expertise.

Dr. David Holt

Doctor Holt was my transplant surgeon. When I heard that he was on the front cover of *Time* magazine, I knew I would be in good hands.

Dr. Holt not only did my kidney transplant, he also operated on my hernia. He is an amazing man. I have the highest respect for this doctor. All of my visits were very interesting and educational. He answered all our questions and gave me a wonderful feeling every time my wife and I visited him.

Thank you from the bottom of my heart, Dr. Holt.

Dr. John Milner

When I first met Dr. Milner, I was very impressed with the way he spoke. With a soft and friendly voice, he greeted me and my wife. Immediately, I knew I was in the best of care. Dr. Milner also operated on me, performing the removal of my native kidneys.

Before the operation, my son Tommy and I met with Dr. Milner in his office. The doctor wanted to prepare me for the operation. He saw what a good attitude I had and was very pleased with me. He said that he wished all his patients were like me.

Dr. Milner told me that first one kidney would be removed, and, a few weeks later, he would remove the other. During the operation, which lasted about six hours, Dr. Milner saw how healthy my organs were, so he took both kidneys out. After the operation, Dr. Milner said he had never seen such healthy organs on a sixty-one-year-old man.

I was very happy and satisfied that the operation was a success. I have the highest respect and admiration for Dr. Milner. I thank you, doctor, for everything.

Dr. John Shea

I've known Dr. Shea since 1992. He was the best neurological surgeon in the country.

I had severe back problems and was rushed to Palos Hospital. The doctor immediately wanted to operate on me. My wife, Jennie, told the doctor that he was too quick to take the knife to me. She wanted a second opinion.

An ambulance took me to Loyola, where I saw Dr. Shea. He said the operation could be done anytime. He suggested physical therapy. He was right.

After a few months I felt great. Then, in 1997, I fell, and I had severe pain shooting down my leg. I was in tears. Dr. Shea told me that the time had come for my surgery. Soon after he operated on me, I felt like a new man again.

When I had my kidney transplant, Dr. Shea came to see me. I was so honored that we embraced each other and he said," I love you, Tom."

I said, "I love you, too, Dr. Shea."

I gave him a copy of my book. Dr. Shea now has Parkinson's disease. I did not know it at the time. But when I saw him a few years later, he told me that he has a good attitude and works out every day. I consider Dr. Shea a good friend. And I will always be there for him. Thank you for everything, Dr. Shea.

Anita Pakrasi, My Transplant Coordinator

The first time I met Anita was when I was being discharged from Loyola Hospital after my kidney transplant. She was explaining to my wife, my daughter, and me my future appointments with the doctors and describing my medications—when and how to take them.

Just listening to the way Anita spoke made me realize how important she would be to ensuring that my kidney continued functioning efficiently. She is very knowledgeable and well-educated in this field. I knew I was in good hands.

Anita knows that I have Parkinson's disease. So, with the other doctors, she has the responsibility of making sure that my medicines will not affect my illness.

I could sense how loving and caring Anita is with not only me, but with all transplant patients. Jennie and I are very satisfied with the way she takes care of me.

Whenever I have questions about my medicines or my kidney, Anita is there to help me. Any medicines prescribed by another doctor have to go through Anita for clearance. Speaking to Anita is just like talking to the doctor.

Anita is a wonderful person, and I hope that in the years to come, she will still be there for me. Thank you, Anita, for everything so far. God bless you.

Father Nick Jonas

I have known Father Nick for many years. He is a wonderful man, dedicated to serving God. By doing this, he is teaching us the laws and the ways of the Christians.

Father Nick has always been there for my family—and especially for me. Father Nick knows how dedicated I am to my workouts. He calls me an inspiration, and that alone makes me want to exercise more. It is Father Nick who believes in me and the way I fight Parkinson's disease like no one else can.

After twelve years with Parkinson's and much praying, I know that Father Nick will always be there—not only for me but my family as well. Besides me, he has all the rest of the parishioners to deal with. God bless you, Father Nick.

About the Author

I have always been and always will be an exercise aficionado. I believe that exercise is mandatory and essential to the human body. I have a master's degree in health, physical education, and exercise physiology. I dissected cadavers to learn how the human body functions.

I not only exercise on a regular basis, but I also play racquetball, golf, ride my mountain bike, practice martial arts, swim, and play backgammon, chess, and Scrabble. Along with several other activities, these are the things I love to do. And I do these activities to the best of my abilities; I strive for perfection.

In the air force, I was among the top out of the sixty-six airmen in basic training. I received the honor of being highly qualified.

When I was discharged from the air force, I decided to go to college. I worked two jobs and went to school full-time. I was advised by the dean of the school not to waste my time and that I would never make it, being married with two children and working two jobs. He even told me that in ten years of being dean, he had never been proven wrong. Although it was very difficult, thanks to my wife's encouragement and support, I persevered.

On the day of graduation, the dean not only apologized to me, but he also praised my educational abilities. It felt great all over.

A few years later, I met someone whom I considered my best friend, Joe Callahan. We had much in common, but he excelled at everything he did. Joe died suddenly in church one day, before his sixty-third birthday. The week before he died, he bench-pressed four hundred pounds three times. He always worked out like he was being rejuvenated. Joe will always be in my heart.

Some years later, I met another man who not only exercises but is a perfectionist in martial arts. His name is John Backshis. John is one of four people in the world who know the seven hundred moves of fighting like twelve animals of Tai Chi. Joe Callahan had a second-degree black belt, I have a fourth degree, and John is a seventh-degree black belt. We practiced for years; we ran, we biked, etc. He is very close to us, and we consider him family.

We all studied under Robert J. Lee, who was considered one of the greatest martial artists of modern times. His unmatched skill and knowledge helped me to be a better person. Thanks to this great man, I can overcome any obstacles or challenges that face me. I, along with about a dozen other black belts, will be forever grateful and indebted to Sensei Lee. He was not only my teacher but a very good friend. To have learned from Robert Lee was not only an experience, but truly an honor as well. I still practice whenever I can. It is a way of life.

I will never forget these three men in my life. Because of their motivation and determination, I am what I am today.

I learned much love from my mother and father. What they taught me, I taught my children. I wish my mother were here today to share in my glory, but I know that her spirit is near me.

I intend to do public speaking on this horrible disease, hoping to inspire and motivate people with all illnesses. I know now that it is my destiny. To help just one person will be rewarding; to help many is God's will.